Table of Con

Preface: How This Book Was Born
Chapter 1: The Champion*slip*
Chapter 2: Conquer Fear by Developing Focus through Mindfulness
Chapter 3: Fearless Flowcharts
Chapter 4: The Champion*slip* Again
About the Authors

Preface

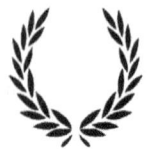

How This Book Was Born

As a parent of a gymnast, I have attended quite a few gymnastics competitions in the past nine years, not knowing how this sport was impacting my young athlete's mind. From the parent point of view, this sport has given my daughter opportunities to become physically and mentally strong. Though this is true, I have also noticed many young gymnasts who are fighting against their fear—of failing, falling, or otherwise being publicly embarrassed—without any coping skills. It is true that many of them feel stuck and lose their confidence. Yet they mask all these difficult emotions and act as if nothing is wrong because they are expected to be strong.

Some coaches say, "Get over it," "Just do it," or, "Don't be scared." I get it. But if these words really worked, most kids wouldn't be nervous in the first place. What if we taught them how to navigate from frantic and desperate thoughts to logical and hopeful thoughts? Conquering fear for trying something new or facing failure in the future comes before mastering physical skills. As a teacher, I have experienced similar frustration in my classroom that the gymnastics coaches might be experiencing as well.

Although my professional training doesn't include specific gymnastics-related physical skills, I know that learning social emotional skills ("SEL" for short) is fundamental for students in order to learn new academic skills in school. Students who can manage their emotions show their resilience in challenging situations, seek resources that are helpful, and initiate problem-solving strategies. Mindfulness is an essential tool that helps students learn focus, self-management, and emotional intelligence. It only makes sense for teachers to teach children what emotions they are experiencing and how to handle their strong emotions when they arise. The mental training makes the students confident and open-minded towards new learning. Understanding and loving yourself can be the starting point of learning. Therefore, it is only logical for teachers to guide students how to do it, and that is what I do in my classroom.

If athletes were to train their minds as tough as they train their physical bodies, they would become champions in any sport. After many years of observing young gymnasts, in addition to my professional educational experience, I've learned that teaching athletes how to be aware of themselves is extremely essential to start training for any sport. In fact, one of the key components of SEL is self-awareness. It must be introduced and practiced daily.

As I found myself contemplating this one evening after dinner, I saw that my daughter Chelsea was working on her middle school narrative essay assignment. She carefully but excitedly carried her laptop to me and exclaimed, "Mom, do you like the title?"

"Champion*slip*."

This word play was brilliant! "Champion Slips in the Championships." Yes, it really happens all the time. And this perfectly summed up Chelsea's own journey to be a champion on her own terms.

I brought up my idea to Chelsea and told her how I wanted to develop something that would help gymnasts conquer their fear. As a result, we created flow charts that any level of athlete can use to navigate their mind when they experience some anxiety during practices, warmups, and competitions. Chelsea agreed to work on this project as a writing partner, a consultant as a gymnast, and a contributor of her original homework essay in this book.

In this book, you will learn:

1. How one teenage gymnast's true voice is spoken towards championship on her own terms,
2. How to build a resilient mind,
3. How to navigate flow charts to conquer fear and self-doubt, and
4. Updates on Chelsea's gymnastics journey.

Chapter 1

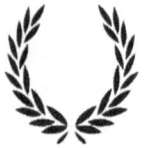

The Champion*slip*

It was a scorching hot afternoon in the summer of 2018 at the Olympic Gymnastics Center in Silverdale, Washington. While hundreds of gymnasts were training as if they were going to compete in the Olympics that day, I was waiting in line, about to do a whip double tuck. I had been trying to perfect this skill before the competition season started so that I could come back from my recent injury.

Towards the end of the season in 2016, I began to notice a slight, dull pain in my right elbow. But I never imagined that it was going to be a serious injury because most gymnasts always had some kind of pain. Luckily, I had hardly ever had serious gymnastics-related injuries until that point. One time, I rolled my ankle while I was jogging during gym class warmups. Another time, I disjointed my pinky knuckle after I caught a football on vacation. During my recovery from both injuries, I had to stay out of gymnastics practice for a couple of weeks, but that was it. Because there had been no significant accident to produce this elbow pain, I didn't even mention it to my parents or coaches. I was so focused on the upcoming Level 8 Regionals. I didn't want to be a "whiner" with small complaints. Nobody really knows about that kind of mental pressure, except gymnasts who have rigorously trained for several years. Gymnastics involves not only the gymnasts themselves, but also coaches and families. We hate disappointing people who support, love, and care about us and our achievements.

As the report of the injury was delayed, the injury worsened. Welcome to the club. I became one of 86,000 gymnasts that year who had an injury and was treated in a medical facility. Finally, after the end of the season, my mother took me to a physical therapist. But even after several sessions of physical therapy, my elbow was still not healed as much as we had hoped.

My physical therapist referred me to the orthopedic doctor to do some x-rays on it. The doctor analyzed the photo of my bone and looked quizzical. He then ordered an MRI scan. Finally, my right elbow was diagnosed with having osteochondritis dissecans, OCD for short. My friend had recently been diagnosed with the same injury. OCD is caused by repetitive stress that commonly appears in the elbow. My friend ended up having surgery, and this possibility scared my parents more than me. For my case, though, at the time, the surgery wasn't a recommended option.

Initially, I was told to stay away from practice for three weeks, but my pain didn't improve as I had wished. Consequently, I had to stay out of almost all meets and championships for two consecutive seasons. During those two long years, I continued to go to the gym, even though I only did conditioning work. I visited Seattle Children's a few times for a second opinion and more MRI scans. Every time we visited the doctor's office, it always came back, "No gymnastics at all." These doctor visits were most frustrating because no matter how many weeks they demanded that I stay out of practice, the pain in my elbow persisted. The good news was that my OCD region was decreasing in size.

Eventually, my mom announced, "Chelsea, we will work together to manage your pain. Let's trust our gut." Her gut told her to rely on Eastern medicine that I wasn't so familiar with. However, my mother grew up with these unique remedies in Japan. She was astonished by how sophisticated our body's natural ability is to heal itself. I started acupuncture treatment regularly and later added maguwart heating. Gradually, my pain lessened. My mother encouraged me to sit with her during her mindfulness meditation. At bedtime, I laid on my back and practiced body scan meditation. With each breath, I guided my attention to each body part, starting at my toes and working up to my head. This exercise relaxed me and I fell asleep while doing a body scan each night. Gradually, I became keen to my pain's severity, duration, and frequency. I began to increase my training time, yet I stopped practicing as soon as I noticed pain. Thankfully, my coaches and I were on the same page and they supported my alternative way of participating in practice.

The process of my healing was a long and painful journey, but I eventually started to get back into routines and competition season.

After missing two competition seasons since the injury, my elbow was finally well enough to resume full-time training. I gained my strength back little by little. To get caught up, my fellow gymnasts and I practiced all of the old and new skills, drills, and conditioning for four hours every day. Our coaches gave us corrections and we were to repeat them until we perfected each skill. I wiped sweat from my forehead with my wristband often during that intense summer training. One after another, we tumbled diagonally across the floor. Slowly, I began to pick up the pace I had prior to my injury. It was clearly my muscle memory. During one particular practice, I was really in the zone, performing every skill with hardly any errors. As I perfectly planted my feet on the bouncy, carpeted floor, my turn was over and I walked up to my coaches for feedback. Instead of giving me any corrections, they told me the plan for this competition season, almost demanding that this was how it was going to be. "Okay, Chelsea. This year we are obviously trying to get you to have three passes. First pass, double back. Second pass, front layout front full. And third pass, one and a half punch front pike. If we don't get the double in time, I will not let you compete with three passes because it's not worth the extra deductions."

I thought to myself, Why are they so determined that I get my double in time? I just got back from my injury! Don't they get that I am not in good shape right now? I don't even have good stamina for three passes!

All I could think about was how I would disappoint them and not meet their expectations. Before I got injured, people used to call me the perfect gymnast because I won so many championships and barely ever made any mistakes. But now, I was always thinking about everything in a negative way and was definitely not confident in myself.

Even though I didn't think I would compete the double on floor, I still worked extremely hard so that I could make everyone happy. It was so typical for me to be under such mental pressure. Champions must get up no matter what. Was I tired of pleasing others with my own performance? No, because I liked the feeling of competing in front of a mesmerized audience. I wished my coaches would have considered how hard it was to maintain a perfect record on difficult skills after a long absence from an injury. At the same time, I wondered where my love of this sport had gone. Was it still in me just like when I started gymnastics?

* * *

My gymnastics journey started unexpectedly, somewhat through a detour. When I was three, as an extremely shy preschooler, my parents first enrolled me in dance lessons. They wanted me to feel pretty and confident in ballet. My mother and I went to the store and looked for a pink leotard, white tights, and soft, pink shoes. Unlike my mother's excitement, I wasn't sure if this was something as fun as what I had already been doing every day with my preschool teacher Margie, like baking bread, climbing willow trees, playing dress up, and painting.

On the day of my first ballet lesson, my Nana showed up and was so proud. She exclaimed, "Oh, Chelsea, look how adorable you are! I will definitely take pictures! Claire, send me yours, too." The ballet studio was large and surrounded by metal bars. We little dancers were directed to sit on the beautifully polished wooden floor. The teacher was a tall, thin woman wearing a tutu. She even had a pretty pink wand in her hand. She began to talk about "stories," something that did not entertain me, although it was connected to ballet. It was long and boring. In fact, some of the girls decided to stand up and wander around the room. My eyes followed them, but my bottom was still glued on the well-polished floor.

Finally, she put her head closely into our little group and announced with a huge grin, "You get to wear your own tutu and a flower crown!" The teacher helped each of us, one by one, pick our very own tutu and flower crown. It wasn't so bad, but not so exciting. I would have rather been playing dress up with a big hat and large high heels in Margie's daycare next to our house. After we were all dressed in our tutus and crowns, we had to sit and listen to the teacher talk… again. Then she passed each of us a magic wand just like hers. There were three dainty strings on the top of the wand. Now this was getting fun. I was ready to do something with this toy.

When we got up, my legs were numb and I felt like I was going to fall straight on my bottom. But I could play. The teacher led the group, and we followed her in a single-file line. We circled the room walking once, running twice, and skipping three times. "Great job, girls! See you next week!" Whhhaaat? Were we done? Yes, it was over. I pulled down my tutu and returned it with the crown and wand, just as the other girls did.

"Chelsea, you did great today! Did you have fun?" My mother asked excitedly. "I can't wait for next time," Nana grinned. I didn't say much except, "It was okay, but I don't like it," very quietly.

The next lesson came. Same routine. Sitting, teacher talking, legs numb. After the lesson, I declared. "I am not going back to ballet." My parents thought I was joking. Even if it were true, they didn't want me to be a quitter at such a young age, so they kept on encouraging me throughout the week. But my mind was firmly set. On the third lesson, I officially quit being a ballerina.

My life went back to normal again for a while. My dad and I walked about 75 steps to Margie's house each morning. I played, ate, and napped there until my mother picked me up. Shortly after I turned four, there was a community invitation for a gymnastics open house in the neighboring town of Port Angeles. Since I quit ballet, my parents wanted me to do something more than daycare and preschool-level activities. Gymnastics was a perfect fit. The most attractive fact, for my parents, was the FREE admission for the event.

When we stepped into the gym, many rambunctious children were already running around the bouncy floor, and some kids were tiptoeing on the high balance beam holding their parent's hand. I was overwhelmed with the size of the facility and the number of random children. That was the most people I had ever seen in one place at one time. The only thing that I was familiar with was three of my friends from daycare! I hesitated a little at first, but my mother took my hand and began to explore all of the different equipment. I bounced on the tumble track. I rolled on the carpeted floor. The floor was not as hard as the ballet studio's. It was bouncy! My dad hoisted my body up onto the high beam. Wow! I was taller than my dad! My mother anxiously reached her arms out, just in case I fell. But I walked down the whole beam by myself! At the end of the open session, the director handed me a registration form for kinder gym classes. This time, I was a little more positive about signing up for the class.

Although open gym was fun, I was still a shy four-year-old in my first class. My body was stuck behind my mom's legs and did not want to move. My hands grabbed my mother's pants so tightly that she couldn't move herself either. "Okay, Chelsea, I will do the class just like you. I want to learn what to do with you," my mother said. She became a "big" student in the circle. We made an imaginative pizza in front of our straddled legs, sprinkling toppings, and it was supposed to be yummy. We moved from station to station, to things like the low bar, short beam, and cheese block. By the end of the class, I had totally forgotten about my mother. My mom became a kinder gym student one more time and then she successfully withdrew from the class. I was now confident to walk into the gym class all by myself.

* * *

While I wasn't sure where my love for gymnastics was, or whether I was still a champion or not, I eventually increased my skill on floor. But it lacked consistency. I still hadn't developed stamina to perform my entire floor routine without falling. Nervous thoughts entered my brain every time it was my turn to perform my floor routine. Everything in my mind was wrapped around the idea of my double back, and I was never quite confident enough to do my routine by myself. It meant my coach stood with his arms crossed in the middle of the floor, watching me flip. His eyes were on me and his hands were ready to spot me, just in case.

The Auburn meet started at 6:30 p.m. It was a late meet, which most people disliked, especially on long, dark, winter days. It would last until 10:30 p.m., including the award ceremony.

Our first event was the vault. Coming back from an elbow injury meant that I had to perform an easier vault routine that didn't have as much impact as other types. I raised my arms up to salute the judges right before I started sprinting, feeling every strike of my feet hitting the ground. I punched the springboard with as much power as I could muster to flip over the vault and land on my feet. My Tsukahara (a style of vault named after Mitsuo Tsukahara, a Japanese male artistic gymnast) was nearly perfect.

Next was the beam. As you might know, the beam requires the balance of a flamingo and the artistry of an elegant butterfly, dancing in the wind. My series—a front aerial into a backflip—went seamlessly. Before I knew it, I was done with my beam routine, and I was able to stay on the whole time.

Floor was the last event, and by then, it was about 9:30 at night. The whole day was building up to this moment and I could feel all of the pressure throughout my whole body. Warmups were good. In fact, since the floor at the meet was bouncier than the floor at our gym, I was able to do my double back easily without a spot. I was ready to go; in about five minutes, it was my time to shine!

I remember my coach telling me that he was only going to stand there just in case something went wrong, but he wasn't planning on spotting me at all. I could hear the crowd cheering in the background as my heart pounded, blood rushing towards my head. My first pass. Round off, whip, double back, I think to myself. I heard my music start and my arms flow to the rhythm. I saw my coach standing there, ready for me to go. I took my first running step, and things started happening fast. I took off for my first flip, and I could hear the wind rush past my ear with a little hum in the crowd.

In an instant, I felt a sharp pain on the right side of my face. Of course, I had fallen during competition. Later, I viewed my performance on video, and I could see that it was a horrendous crash on the right side of my face and my ankle. My body was crouched on the floor for one second, and suddenly, I pushed myself up and proceeded to the corner of the floor. No wonder I could barely see out of my right eye.

At that moment, I was about to stop my floor routine, as any other gymnast would have done, but the adrenaline rushed through my whole body, commanding me to complete the routine. No one expected me to keep going after such an agonizing fall. Even just watching it brought the audience pain. Despite the pain on my right side, I continued my routine and ended up making all of my other passes, as if nothing had happened.

After my routine was over, I walked to my coach. She started telling me that everything happens for a reason. This was her way of telling me that I was so strong for finishing my routine. "Falling is not a weakness. Completing the whole routine after your fall is a strength." Did I hear my coach's words right? I thought that if what she said was true, I would become even stronger without a fall at the next meet.

After the hugs and the talks with my coaches and some of my teammates, my eyes filled up with tears. The adrenaline was gone and my normal state of mind returned. However, I was not sad or disappointed. I wasn't quite sure why I cried for so long.

Looking back, there was nothing to be ashamed about. I worked super hard to perfect that skill, and I did. That was only about two seconds of my life, and I most certainly wouldn't let it bring me down. Champions slip. It's okay to fall. Getting up makes you a champion. Even though I didn't get a first place at this meet, I knew I was still a champion inside and I was proud.

The next day, I woke up and felt a sharp pain in my ankle. I realized that I injured myself when I landed so badly. My ankle was as swollen as a baseball and it felt like it was clamped in a vise-like grip, not able to move. My right eye had a dark bruise on it, like after a fistfight.

But despite all of the outward pain, I knew this experience would just build me into a better and more hardworking gymnast. You would think champions win because they flip most elegantly. But champions become champions after they slip most painfully. The pain makes champions stronger. The resilience against adversity is the unique strength that true champions possess. The championship happens in a true champion's heart every time she slips. This mental strength is what I work on every day because I call myself a champion.

Chapter 2

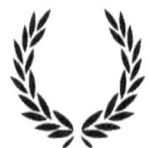

Conquer Fear by Developing Focus through Mindfulness

We have to point out that when a gymnast is at a competition, especially a big one (state, regional, or national championships, elite qualifier meets, etc.), her mind is easily overwhelmed by the atmosphere and fellow competitors. It is so important for her to stay calm by developing self-awareness while in those chaotic surroundings.

Instead of overwhelming herself or being distracted, a gymnast can rehearse how many times and how she succeeded at her difficult skills in practice. That is the driving reason to be calm. There is nothing to be afraid of if she is able to focus on what she can do during practice.

Additionally, easy techniques like this one-minute breathing exercise will help calm the nerves. Slowly breathe in through the nose and pause for three seconds. Then breathe out from the mouth, like a big sigh. At the third breath out, one minute is up.

Mindfulness comes in handy in these situations when the gymnast practices it daily; this simple exercise can be done independently, without any guidance. In a daily mindfulness practice, individual gymnasts can learn what to focus on, when to focus, and how to focus by managing through their emotions. Just like with physical skills, practicing daily mindfulness helps athletes develop self-awareness and learn how to accept any outcome, visualize their success, and be kind in competitive sports. At a big competition, you may say, "It's okay to be nervous." And then you could add, "I have a tool to calm down. Breathe in and breathe out." How cool would that be?

Why Daily Mindfulness Practice?

Mindful meditation is getting popular in sports, especially since many professional and collegial athletes have used it to obtain amazing results. Why? Because every competition requires the ability to focus. The ability to focus is something you can strengthen with mindfulness practice.

The Seattle Seahawks head coach, Pete Carol, publicly announced that meditation was one of the major keys to the 2016 Super Bowl victory. The team constantly practiced to be focused on what was important under the extreme pressure.

In addition to his super natural talent and work ethic, LeBron James' successful athletic career can also be credited to his daily private meditation at home. In the 2012 NBA Playoffs, his meditation to refocus during the timeout was viewed by thousands of fans on television.

Misty May-Treanor and Kerri Walsh agreed that their daily practice of yoga and visual meditation contributed hugely to their three consecutive Summer Olympic gold medal championships in beach volleyball.

Why do they have to meditate? They are already good at their sports, you might be asking. I will return the exact same question back to you. Why do you think they practice mindfulness? Because they think they are already good at their sports?

Fighting Against Fear

In 2012, Cincinnati gymnastics coach Mary Lee Tracy brought two elite gymnasts, Lexi and Amelia, to the gymnastics clinic in Eastern Washington. All young participants were excited to see and get to practice with special elites who were trying to make it onto the Olympic team. They all admired these elite gymnasts' flawless movements and were almost jealous of their level of talent.

After the break, Mary Lee started to talk about sports psychology. "Raise your hand if you are scared of some skills." All the girls shot up their hands, including Lexi and Amelia.

Mary Lee continued, "You would think these elite gymnasts don't have any fears and everything is so easy. You are wrong. They are scared, too. But they know when they are scared and what they have to do to refocus when they are scared."

Takeaways from this locally held session included learning how to notice the emotion you are feeling and to refocus your attention back to what you are doing at that moment. I had never heard of the word "mindfulness" at this time, but thinking back, it was so evident that gymnasts and all other athletes must strengthen their awareness in order to be successful in their career.

As we all witnessed, Team USA dominated in the women's gymnastics in the 2016 Rio Olympic Games. There is no doubt that all U.S. Olympians are talented, but not very many people recognized that these extremely skillful athletes also struggle. Robert Andrews, a sports psychology coach who worked with Simone Biles, recalls her mental struggles, according to Alyssa Roenick in an ESPN article from August 2016. Andrews, a well-trained and experienced sports psychology coach, was patient when he saw Biles. And he listened. Andrews' advice was simple and clear each time: "Whatever happens, you choose how to respond, and the more mindful you are, the better choices you make."

Laurie Hernandez' coach Maggie Haney contacted Andrews to help her gymnast when she read about Andrews' work with Biles. Hernandez learned a simple breathing technique to help her relax. Before each rotation, this young gymnast would put her right hand on her stomach, close her eyes, and take a deep breath. This exact breathing routine of Laurie Hernandez was seen before each routine during the Olympic Trials.

As the competition gets intense, young athletes must obtain the tools to stay calm and sustain their confidence in their skills. Mindfulness can be an extremely effective tool to help conquer an athlete's fear and doubt. Mental pressure caused by the high intensity of physical trainings can be managed by implementing a daily mindfulness practice.

As Robert Andrews shared, "A wobble on beam might shake Simone's confidence for a few seconds, but her belief in her ability will remain rock solid."

Successful Athletics Career

Needless to say, every athlete cannot be an Olympian, even though it can be everybody's goal. So, let's talk about what the definition of success in sports is for you. What makes a young athlete feel successful in everyday workouts?

First, having a long-term goal or vision—wanting to be on the Olympic team for instance—is fantastic. Unfortunately, it is true that, even if they have a big vision, many athletes have a difficult time taking and maintaining focused action towards it, beyond just saying that they have a goal. In other words, they don't necessarily work on achieving their long-term goal. In fact, creating a long-term goal and maintaining focus on it are both very challenging tasks, even for adults. Young adults need appropriate guidance on this for sure.

Let's say not having a long-term goal for now is okay because as they build their confidence and successes on daily practices at the gym, young athletes will be able to eventually create a clear vision of their future. At this point, though, all athletes must be fully committed to their sport if they desire to experience success at any level. A coach's advice will help only when the gymnast desires to succeed. When you seek success, you must remember to work hard on your part and be patient; it takes time.

Daily Success with the Resilience Cycle

The Japanese proverb "always rise after a fall" tells an important lesson for gymnasts, literally and inferentially. Its original wording is "seven falls eight ups." You might think, "Why eight ups and not seven?" It is a clever trick. It's not bad that you fall seven times and try again by getting up exactly the same number of falls. The eighth up is the bonus: new learning. Instead of doing something over and over the same way, each time you fall, you reflect on the falling experience and adjust for what you want to accomplish. That reflection process makes the next fall more meaningful, and you are most likely improving. Or you are going to stick instead of falling! This is the number one reason you don't have to worry about falling.

This reflection process applies to the "Resilience Cycle." Establishing resilience is essential because gymnastics is a physically and mentally tough sport. You chose this sport because the challenge of it would give you a huge reward in your performance by overcoming hardships. So, first, pat yourself on the back! Then, make sure your mind is always ready with your body for practice each day. You don't need to follow the Resilience Cycle in written form, but instead, you can remember it in your mind and utilize it everyday practice for your success. Remember, each small, successful moment will build up to form your long-term vision.

The Resilience Cycle

1. Have Goals/Plans

After a coach's instruction, take a big breath. Then repeat to yourself the skill and the drills in each progression that you are working on next for 20 minutes. What should the successful outcome look like in each drill? Leaps? Sticks? How to use a certain part of your body? Number of accuracies? Be specific. Make sure you understand 100% what the coach tells you. If you are not clear, ask!

2. Work Intentionally

Time is money. Don't waste. Keep working. Focus on certain tips each time your coach gives them to you. Remember to breathe before and after each try. If you are stuck, take a deep breath to refocus on today's goal and plan. Nobody sets your goal for you. (Would you ask your friend, "Can you please go to the bathroom for me"? No! You are the one who needs to go to the bathroom and take care of business!) You are responsible for your own success.

3. Allow Mistakes/Falls

This is a simple fact, yet people often forget. No matter what level you are on, gymnasts fall. You are training yourself to stick more consistently because "the stick" creates a beautiful and accomplishing moment. Perhaps your goal today is to stick on the dismount. It is because landing is challenging. Be kind to yourself. Allow yourself to fall. In the process of achieving success, falling happens.

4. Reflect on Success and Mistakes

Although falling happens, don't let it happen without thought. When you fall, it is a learning opportunity. Remember, seven falls and eight ups. Not only do you need to get up and try again, but you also need to make it intentional. Analyze how the fall happened and what you should do next time. That's a plus one bonus point.

5. Turn Mistakes into Your Next Goal

During the drills, your turn comes quickly. Once you identify your mistakes and your coach gives you corrections, you have your next goal. Listen to your coach carefully and take three big breaths. The next gymnast might be waiting for her turn; you can do this process fairly quickly. If you are not sure what you are doing or what your coach is talking about, ask! And remember to appreciate them for their support.

The Resilience Cycle

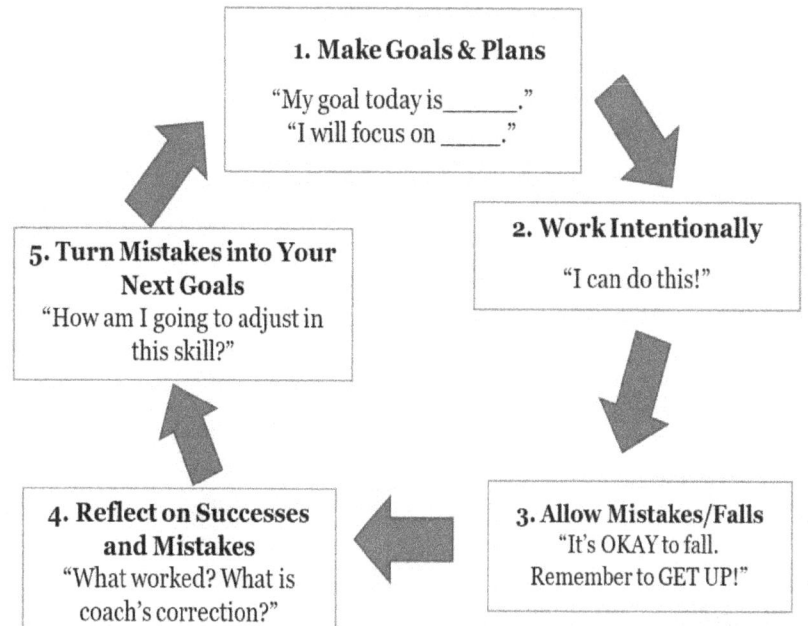

Break Through the Wall of Fear

It's possible to feel fear when you think about what happened in the past or when you try to predict something that might happen in the future. You might be scared of the bar because you were injured last time. You might be afraid of your coach because she/he yelled at you yesterday. It's reasonable to expect something similar to happen on your next turn based upon these past experiences. That's why athletes must improve their focusing skills instead of being scared and anxious.

When your focus is in the moment, you are on the Resilience Cycle. As you start a daily mindfulness meditation practice, you can improve your focus level and its duration gradually. Mindfulness will help you become more aware of what's happening in you and your surroundings. Instead of reacting to your negative thoughts or strong emotions (sabotaging the practice or pouting in the corner), it will help you navigate back to a calm state of mind where you can think logically and make wise choices (e.g., come back to the Resilience Cycle). Fear can protect you from danger, but if you have a goal to achieve, you must learn how to tame this emotion when it's necessary.

Fear Mechanism

When you experience fear, your body responds accordingly because of a part of your brain called the amygdala, which sends a signal to your sympathetic nervous system to take control. It physically affects your body: your pupils dilate, your breathing gets fast and shallow, your heart pumps faster, and your gut goes inactive. The amygdala is famously known as "fight, flight, and freeze." In ancient times, the amygdala was very helpful in protecting our ancestors from dangers like unpredictable animal attacks, for instance. Imagine walking on a trail and seeing a cougar suddenly jump out from a bush in front of you. Your body freezes. That is how our ancestors survived their harsh environment. There were so many dangers they had to protect themselves from every day. Thankfully, in our era, we don't have to deal with protecting ourselves from cougars in our daily lives. Although our environment has changed and technology has improved over time, the amygdala still lives in our brain, looking for the time it will be needed.

When you remember the last fall from the bar, your amygdala might react to make you feel uncomfortable. It gives the sympathetic nervous system the fight, flight, and freeze signal, and you will then lose your focus. That is the wall you must break through.

Stimulate Your PFC

The great news is that our brain has more than the amygdala. Touch your forehead. That is the place where your prefrontal cortex (PFC) lives. When the PFC is activated, it signals to the parasympathetic nervous system. Unlike the sympathetic nervous system, the parasympathetic nervous system relaxes your body. The PFC supports activities like planning, organizing, strategizing, paying attention, remembering details, and managing time and space. When the PFC is activated, the amygdala quiets down. In other words, you gain your focus back instead of freaking out with fear. And one simple function in your body can stimulate the PFC. Your breaths.

A PFC that is stimulated through mindfulness can develop the aspects of well-being, according to author Daniel Siegel (*The Mindful Brain*, 2007). They include body regulation, self-awareness, emotional regulation, and fear modulation, which can all be seen in the gymnastics world. Body regulation is when balance and coordination are maintained between the acceleration and brakes of the nervous system. It is essential for a gymnast to maintain an appropriate energy level (not extremely high or too low) during gymnastics training and competitions. Self-awareness includes our own sense of ourselves and our ability to visualize a positive future. The dysregulated emotion causes overwhelmed emotional chaos, which would lead to stagnation or depression. When emotion is regulated, life has vitality and meaning. The stimulated PFC also modulates our fear. This promotes our ability to calm, soothe, or even unlearn our own fears.

As you can see, we all have a PFC. And if we stimulate it, we can conquer our fear and improve our focus at each moment. You are the one who is in charge of your PFC!

Breaths: Your Super Power

Now, you are probably wondering how to stimulate the PFC. Before we go over that, you have to remember that it will take time. Do you remember how long it took you to do your first kip? You worked on it over and over, every single day. Then, one day, you mastered it, and since then, this skill has gotten easier. You are now able to swift your body up on the bar with minimum effort. Practicing mindfulness is similar. You must commit to your practice every day. You will become more aware gradually; however, it's even harder to notice the improvement because your brain stays inside. When you notice that you are sticking with the Resilience Cycle, that is an improvement. When you notice that you are frustrated, that is an improvement. Why? When you notice your negative emotions sneaking in, you are able to pause and refocus. That is the skill we are about to improve. Our secret weapon lives way closer than you might think. It is in your body. Your breaths.

Add Mindfulness Meditation as a Regular Routine

As you build stronger muscles, adding mindfulness to your regular routine will also build a stronger brain muscle, which will clear the accessible path to the PFC before the amygdala reacts. Our goal is to start a short mindfulness routine, increase the time little by little, and eventually, maintain 10 to 15 minutes of independent mindful practice each day. Although mindfulness meditation doesn't require specific objects in the practice, tangible objects, some movements, and/or vocal guidance might be helpful if you are very new to this. You may choose what is best for you to continue towards the goal of an independent 10- to 15-minute practice.

To build the strength in your muscle and mind, you can follow a six-week plan. During this time, you can use the journal that I provide in the appendix of this book. This journal will support your strong mind journey during and after the six-week plan. I highly recommend continuing to the advanced journal for 10 to 15 minutes of independent mindfulness practice. Reviewing your old journal entries often gives you important information and insights that you might have missed in the past.

Before jumping into the practice, find a regular space where you can sit straight on the floor or on a chair. As we practice "focusing," the spinal cord is straight so that your body is not too relaxed (sleep). A mindfulness exercise can be short, but needs to be consistent: do it every day. If you are inspired by the stories of Laurie Hernandez and Simone Biles, you are ready!

Work with an Accountability Partner

Although an accountability partner is optional, it is very effective if you are very serious about becoming a champion. Sharing your goal and progress is not only fun, but it makes you more responsible on the tasks that you are accomplishing. So, work on your mindfulness with your partner. You and your partner don't need to have the same goals or even have goals in the same field, but you should both want to accomplish something. Think of whom you could ask to be your partner. Your best friend? Coach? Or even your mom!

Meet up with your accountability partner once a week to share your goals and report how you did in the previous week. Goals can be centered around your gymnastic skills and mindfulness practice. Journaling is also helpful to keep you accountable on your task completion.

Just like your coach gives you corrections in practice, someone needs to monitor your progress in your mental training. That person is YOU! Reflecting on your own practice will help you improve your skills, which will lead to an increase in your self-confidence. Feel free to use the journals I created (*Appendix A and B*). If you have a partner, recording and sharing your progress (ups and downs) will impact the mental strength of both you and your partner. Be committed!

Week 1: One-Minute Practice

The goal for Week 1 is to be aware of the length of one minute. One minute can feel long or short, depending on what you are doing. The awareness of the minute increases your consciousness, appreciation of the moment, and hopes for the upcoming practice in the next few weeks. There are several ways that you can practice. You can choose one method to do the same throughout the week, or you can do a new activity each day to enjoy some variety.

1. Notice Your Breaths

Put your hand on your chest or belly. Breathe in through your nose slowly. Hold for three seconds. Then breathe out slowly through your mouth like a sigh. Hold for three seconds. Repeat three times. That's about one minute.

2. Glitter Water Bottle

You need to make a glitter bottle for this practice. Put a tablespoon of glitter in an empty, clear, half-gallon bottle. Then fill it with water until it is about 4/5 full. Seal the lid tightly and shake it. As the glitter settles down, intentionally take big breaths. When it is all settled on the bottom, it has been about one minute.

3. Pipe Cleaner & Three Beads

Put a pipe cleaner through three beads one at a time. Tie both ends of the pipe cleaner like a circle. Slowly breathe in and out as you move one bead around the circle. Then, move each bead back with slow breaths. When all three beads come back, it's about one minute.

4. Yoga Movement (Standing Option)

Stand up straight. Swipe both arms and both hands to meet above your head. Bring both arms down to touch your toes. Repeat three times, which will take you about one minute.

5. Exercise Ball Lift (Standing Option)

You can use a physical ball or pretend ball. Squat to pick up the ball and slowly bring it up above your head. Sway right and left. Slowly bring it down. Repeat three times; that will be about one minute.

6. Finger Valley and Mountain

Open your left hand until all fingers are extended. Touch the tip of your thumb with your right index finger. As your right index finger slowly traces down from the thumb and up to the left index finger, remember to breathe consciously. Continue to trace up and down until you reach your pinky. Do the same motions backwards until your right index finger comes back to the tip of your thumb. Switch your hands and repeat. When both hands are done, it's been about one minute.

7. Guess One Minute

Sit up straight but comfortably. As soon as you set a timer for one minute, close your eyes and start breathing slowly. Open your eyes when you guess the one minute is up. How many seconds were you off by? You must be really close.

Monitor Your Progress

Take some notes in your journal to be more accountable. Keep and review your activities on the **Strengthen Mind and Muscle to Conquer Fear Journal** (*Appendix A*). Reflection is a big part of mental practice, like your coach's corrections. Only this time, you find your strengths and areas to improve by analyzing the records. At the end of the week, review your practice and record it. Prepare to share the results with your partner. The best part of having a partner is encouraging each other and celebrating together!

Meet Up with Your Accountability Partner

Check in with your accountability partner to share your experiences. A weekly meeting benefits both of you and keeps you accountable. You can meet up with your accountability partner in person (the best!), but simply sharing the progress by texting and celebrating with emojis are not bad ideas. While your daily practice happens on your own time and at your own pace, sharing your experiences with someone you trust who may have similar goals enriches your experiences. Be open and honest. Try not to judge each other's progress with thoughts like, "She is doing better than me," or, "I didn't do as much as I was supposed to do because I was too busy." In fact, when you start making excuses, stop for a second. Think about why you started this practice with your partner. You want to improve, right? True champions accept the facts as they are and investigate how to make things more efficient for next time. Previous experiences are only a baseline for the next step. Keep that in mind and have some active discussions with your partner.

Some conversation starters include the following:

- Which activities have you tried?
- What was the highest point of your athletic training this week?
- What skills are you going to work on next week?

Agree to listen to your partner's experiences and give some feedback (compliments, questions, and suggestions) from your heart. To make this routine more fun, you can create a celebration dance to do at the end of the meeting.

Week 2: Two-Minute Practice

Choose one activity a day from last week's list. This week, you are going to double your mindfulness practice. In order to double a minute, simply double the number of trials for each activity. For instance, instead of doing "Notice Your Breath" three times, do it six times. This should not be a big problem if you are already a gymnast. If you find that doubling the time is challenging, try a standing position or movement options. Another alternative can be to set a timer for one minute, just like Week 1. Then relax for a few seconds and set the timer for another minute to try a different activity. Either way, you will double your practice. You can often find solutions in your creativity.

Meet Up with Your Accountability Partner

Prepare your Week 2 reflection on the **Strengthen Mind and Muscle to Conquer Fear Journal** *(Appendix A)* for the meeting. What was hard for you this week? What went well? What caused your results this week? How are they the same or different compared to Week 1? You can jot down some of your thoughts before you meet up with your accountability partner.

Now it is time to check in with your accountability partner to share the summary of your week:

- Which activities have you tried?
- What was the highest point of your athletic training this week?
- When were you scared?
- What did you do when you were scared?
- What skills are you going to work on next week?

Don't forget about your celebration dance that you created. What is your celebration emoji?

Week 3: Three-Minute Practice

Welcome to Week 3! There is nothing to worry about if you already completed Weeks 1 and 2. What you will do is choose one activity a day from the Week 1 list and double it just like last week. Only this time, set a timer for an extra minute at the end of the practice. Sit up straight, close your eyes, and visualize one gymnastics skill that you want to work on today. Take a big deep breath in and out. Start from the beginning, like a shadow practice; only this time, visualize in your mind as many details as possible. What part of the body do you need to use the most? How is the grip? How can you pick up the momentum? Like a movie, let yourself go through the drill or a completed skill in your mind. When you are done, it will have been about three minutes.

Notice your body's sensations and emotions at the end of each practice session. In what body part do you feel the most sensation? How is your energy level? How is your pleasantness?

Meet Up with Your Accountability Partner

You will find this week's share amusing because your partner, too, will share what skill she was visualizing. Your partner's experience might lead to a breaking point. Chances are that your partner's experience can be the breakthrough on some skills that you might be struggling with too. Similarly, your experience can help your partner. After you listen to your partner's experience, you can give her your honest feedback. As you are open with your experience, both of you can empower each other. What do you feel after the meeting? It is a great practice to be aware of your body and mind.

Week 4: Five-Minute Practice with Guidance Recording

One way to increase your mindful meditation practice time is to use applications on your mobile phone or online. If you successfully completed the first three weeks, guided meditation on an app is something new and simple enough to apply. There are so many mindfulness meditation apps for athletes. Simply Google it and find the best fit for you. My favorite is Smiling Mind (https://www.smilingmind.com.au/). I have used this app for personal practice, children's practice, classroom practice, and sports. You can choose a five-minute mindful meditation practice from the app and follow the directions provided. If you are working with young athletes in an elementary school, I recommend the Smiling Mind program for kids. Surprisingly, five minutes will pass very quickly.

Another alternative is to continue to choose activities from Week 1 and extend the time. For example, set a timer for three minutes to do activities from the list and use the next two minutes for visualization.

Whatever you choose, you are going to challenge yourself to complete five minutes of mindfulness practice. It is huge; however, it is not hard at this point. You are strengthening your focus by consistent practice, just as you have been training to improve your gymnastics skills since you were young. Give yourself credit for your hard work. You are becoming a champion on your own terms!

Meet Up with Your Accountability Partner

Share your experience with the guided meditation practice or alternative practice of your choice. The end of Week 4 means that you and your partner committed and completed a daily mindfulness practice for ONE MONTH! That's a great accomplishment! In addition to the celebration, exchange your appreciation for being each other's partner for the last four weeks. Gratitude will become an important ingredient in your championship journey.

- Are this week's activities similar or different to the previous practice?
- How did you feel during practice?
- How do you feel right now?
- Did you notice something (body sensations or emotions) when you took a deep breath during practice?

Week 5: Ten-Minute Practice with Guidance Recording

As the challenge is getting more intense, it is important for you to choose your options on how to organize your 10-minute practice this week. A longer mindfulness meditation will help develop a keener and deeper level of self-awareness. In other words, you would notice small physical and emotional shifts more often. When you notice these changes, your PFC helps you to make logical decisions instead of "fight or flight" fear responses from the amygdala.

Option 1: Stick with the five-minute guidance program from your app from Week 4 and combine the Week 2 two-minute practice and the Week 3 three-minute practice.

Option 2: Find a 10-minute guidance program from your app and apply it in your practice.

Option 3 (advanced): Set a timer for 10 minutes, close your eyes, and count your breath up to 10. When you reach 10, count back to 1. If you become distracted and lose count, simply start over. At the end of the practice, pay attention to your energy level and pleasantness.

Option 4 (advanced): Set a timer for 10 minutes, just like Option 3. The only difference is to visualize your skills that you are working on instead of counting your breaths. Focus on your body sensation during the practice.

Option 5 (advanced): This is a combination of Options 3 and 4. Count your breaths from 1 to 10, and then visualize your skills. When you complete one routine in the visualization, bring your attention back to your breath and start counting them again. When it reaches to 10, visualize the skill again. Be curious about what is happening in each moment. At the end of the practice, take notes in your journal about any particular body sensations on certain skills and emotions that came along.

Meet Up with Your Accountability Partner

Because of the uniqueness of this week's practice, the conversation with your accountability partner should be fun. Be curious about what your partner experienced. How many days did you complete a full 10-minute practice? Do you feel more independent? Did you notice something different during the practice? How did you respond to the fear when you noticed it at the gym during practice? The conversation might be more active during this session. Be sure to respect each other's turn by not interrupting. When you are listening, focus on just listening, even if you are too excited to share your experiences. You will have your own turn. Giving full attention to each other creates a foundation of mutual respect and trust.

- Which option did you try?
- How did you feel during your mindfulness practice?
- When did you take a deep breath during athletic practice?

Week 6: 10-15-Minute Practice with/without Guidance Recording

In the final week, set your timer for 10 or 15 minutes, sit up straight, and practice your focus on one thing during each session. You can focus on 1) your breaths, 2) sounds around you, 3) your stomach rising and falling, 4) do a scan of your body, 5) think of a person you appreciate, or 6) visualize one of your routines at competition.

Whenever you are distracted, simply bring your attention back to what you are focusing on during today's practice. Allow yourself to get distracted because that is what your mind does naturally. When you notice and bring your attention back, you are strengthening your PFC. Over six weeks, your neuroplasticity will have shifted semi-permanently (Anthony Warren, CEO of BreatheSimple, 2017). Your mind used to translate fear into freaking out or shutting down. Now, your mind will translate fear into a pause for breathing because of the six weeks of mindfulness practice. Taming your fear is another name for having a strong mind. When your mind is calm and clear, you are one step closer to winning a championship!

Meet Up with Your Accountability Partner

Time to celebrate with the victory dance or heart-eyed emoji! You and your partner completed one full week of independent mindfulness practice for 10-15 minutes each day, just like LeBron James! After completing six weeks of mindfulness meditation, you will have proven to yourself your commitment and passion for the sport. Your foundation has just been established. It is up to you if you want to actively sustain your strength or come back to the practice as needed. You and your partner now have some decisions to make moving forward, depending on your definition of "champion."

Option 1: Say goodbye to your partner for now and meet up in a month or two. If you feel confident to carry on with independent practice, this option is the best, especially with your advanced journal in *Appendix B*. In a month, you will be able to share more drastic accomplishments with each other.

Option 2: If the two of you feel that it's beneficial to meet every week, continue your 10-minute independent practice daily and meet once per week. It is absolutely okay to do. The **Advanced Strengthen Mind and Muscle to Conquer Fear Journal** *(Appendix B)* will be fruitful to use during your conversations in the following weeks. You can also find a different partner, if you want. In many cases, some people feel more secure having someone by their side who understands what they are doing.

Option 3: Commit to your independent practice exclusively on your own without a journal. This is the way that most adults practice mindfulness. However, I recommend that young gymnasts complete the **Advanced Journal** (*Appendix B*) with their independent mindfulness practice. This way, you can refer to your journal when you need to in the future.

Guide to Strengthen Mind and Muscle to Conquer Fear Journal

Each row of the journal is organized per week. If you complete a weekly mindfulness task seven days a week, it means 100%. Roughly calculate five days as 75%, three days as 50%, and one day as 25%. In the beginning of the week, you fill out your major gymnastics skills (drills) that you are working on during that week in the "Skill Goals" column. At the end of the week, fill out "Accomplished Skills" or drills. Use your own words to describe your experiences in the "Observation and Conversation" column. What were you afraid of this week? Did you notice some moments when you took a breath? As you specify each event, you can focus on the area where you need help or resources that would assist in managing your internal needs.

Appendix A: Strengthen Mind and Muscle to Conquer Fear Journal

Week	Mindfulness Goal	Skill Goals (Day 1)	Accomplished Skills (Day 7)	Observation&Conversation Notice Fear? Take a Breath?
1	One Minute ○ 100% ○ 75% ○ 50% ○ 25%			
2	Two Minutes ○ 100% ○ 75% ○ 50% ○ 25%			
3	Three Minutes ○ 100% ○ 75% ○ 50% ○ 25%			
4	Five Minutes ○ 100% ○ 75% ○ 50% ○ 25%			
5	Ten Minutes ○ 100% ○ 75% ○ 50% ○ 25%			
6	Independent 10-15 minutes ○ 100% ○ 75% ○ 50% ○ 25%			

- Check a bubble each week to indicate how many mindfulness tasks you accomplished: 7 days = 100%, 5-6 days = 75%, 3-4 days = 50%, and 1-2 days = 25%.
- Matching Skill Goals and Accomplished Skills means you have been focused!
- Jot down something you have noticed during the practice and conversation with your accountability partner. Reflection stimulates your PFC.

Appendix B: Advanced Mind and Muscle to Conquer Fear Journal

Week	Mindfulness Goal	Skill Goals (Day 1)	Accomplished Skills (Day 7)	Observation&Conversation Notice Fear? Take a Breath?
7	Independent 10-15 Minutes ○ 100% ○ 75% ○ 50% ○ 25%			
8	Independent 10-15 Minutes ○ 100% ○ 75% ○ 50% ○ 25%			
9	Independent 10-15 Minutes ○ 100% ○ 75% ○ 50% ○ 25%			
10	Independent 10-15 Minutes ○ 100% ○ 75% ○ 50% ○ 25%			
11	Independent 10-15 Minutes ○ 100% ○ 75% ○ 50% ○ 25%			
12	Independent 10-15 Minutes ○ 100% ○ 75% ○ 50% ○ 25%			

- Check a bubble each week to indicate how many mindfulness tasks you accomplished: 7 days = 100%, 5-6 days = 75%, 3-4 days = 50%, and 1-2 days = 25%.
- Matching Skill Goals and Accomplished Skills means you have been focused!
- Jot down something you have noticed during the practice and conversation with your accountability partner. Reflection stimulates your PFC.

Chapter 3

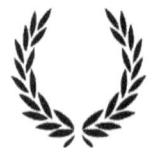

Fearless Flowcharts

On the next few pages, you will find Fearless Flowcharts. No matter how confident you are in practice, "not sure" moments happen unexpectedly. The good news is that you now have a tool to help you refocus. You are learning how to use it. When you notice an icky feeling arise in your stomach, pause and take a deep breath.

If your confidence still hides deep inside of you, take a look at one of the Fearless Flowcharts. You might feel more relaxed by creating an image of your fear through the chart. You might have your own self-talk or other paths that make more sense to you. Soon, your focus will be on your goals and plans in the Resilience Cycle.

Remember, your mind wanders. You have been training through mindfulness how to notice when it happens and how to bring your focus back to where it should be. The Fearless Flowcharts are another tool that will lead you back on track.

Before Practice: Have You Had Some Snacks?

Use this flow chart when practice starts in 20 minutes, but you don't feel like going…

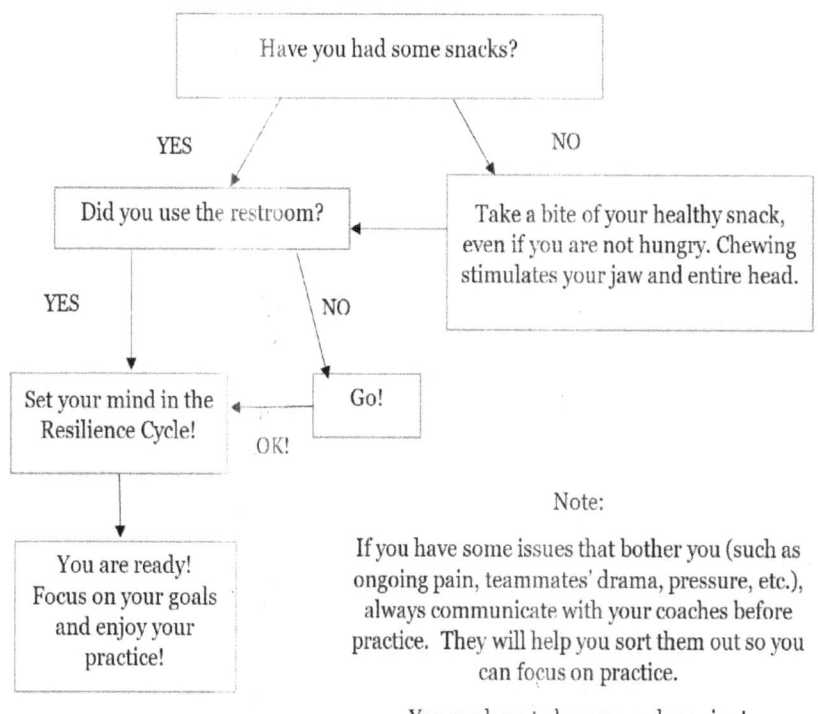

Note:

If you have some issues that bother you (such as ongoing pain, teammates' drama, pressure, etc.), always communicate with your coaches before practice. They will help you sort them out so you can focus on practice.

You are here to become a champion!

During Practice: Are You Afraid of Doing a Skill?

Use this flow chart when you are in doubt about what you have done in previous practices. Remember, gymnastics is a mental game. The tougher the mind, the more accurate the skills.

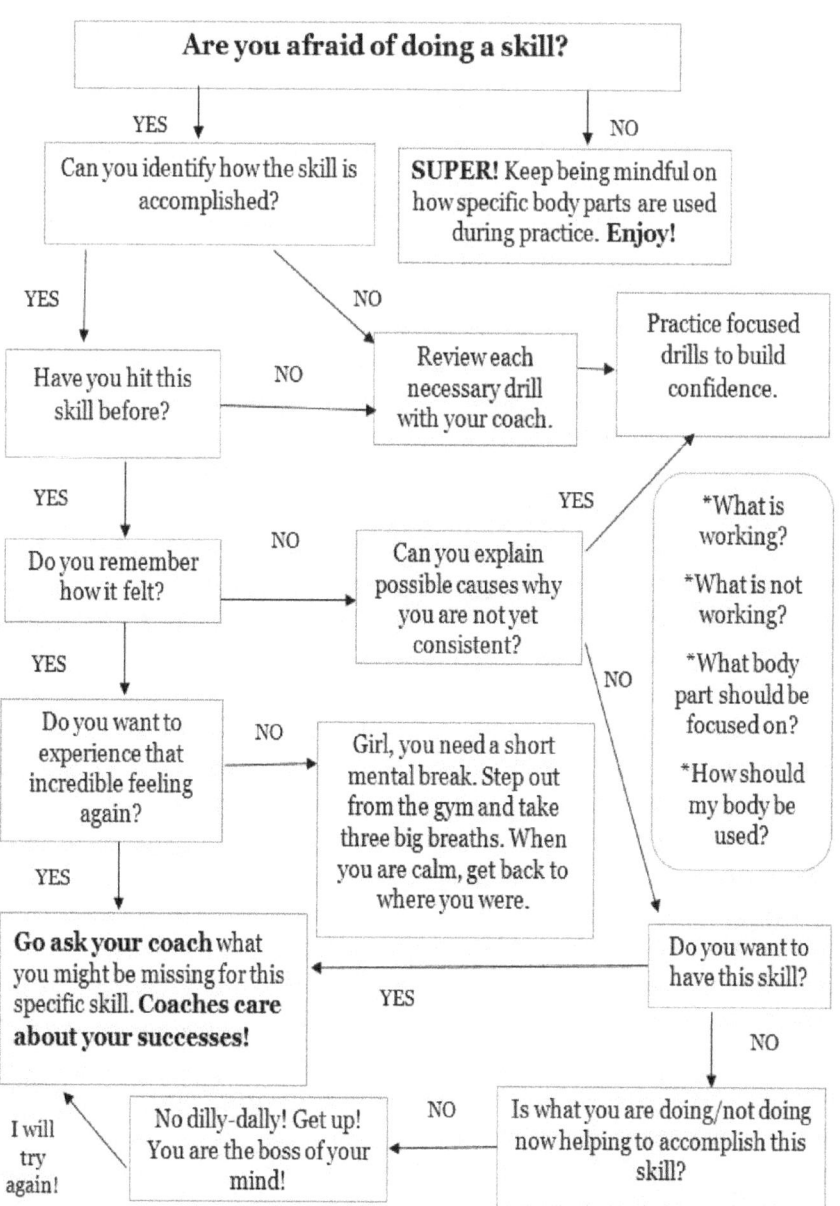

A Week Before the Meet: Are You Ready for This Meet?

Use this flow chart when you are nervous about an upcoming meet. *What am I afraid of?*

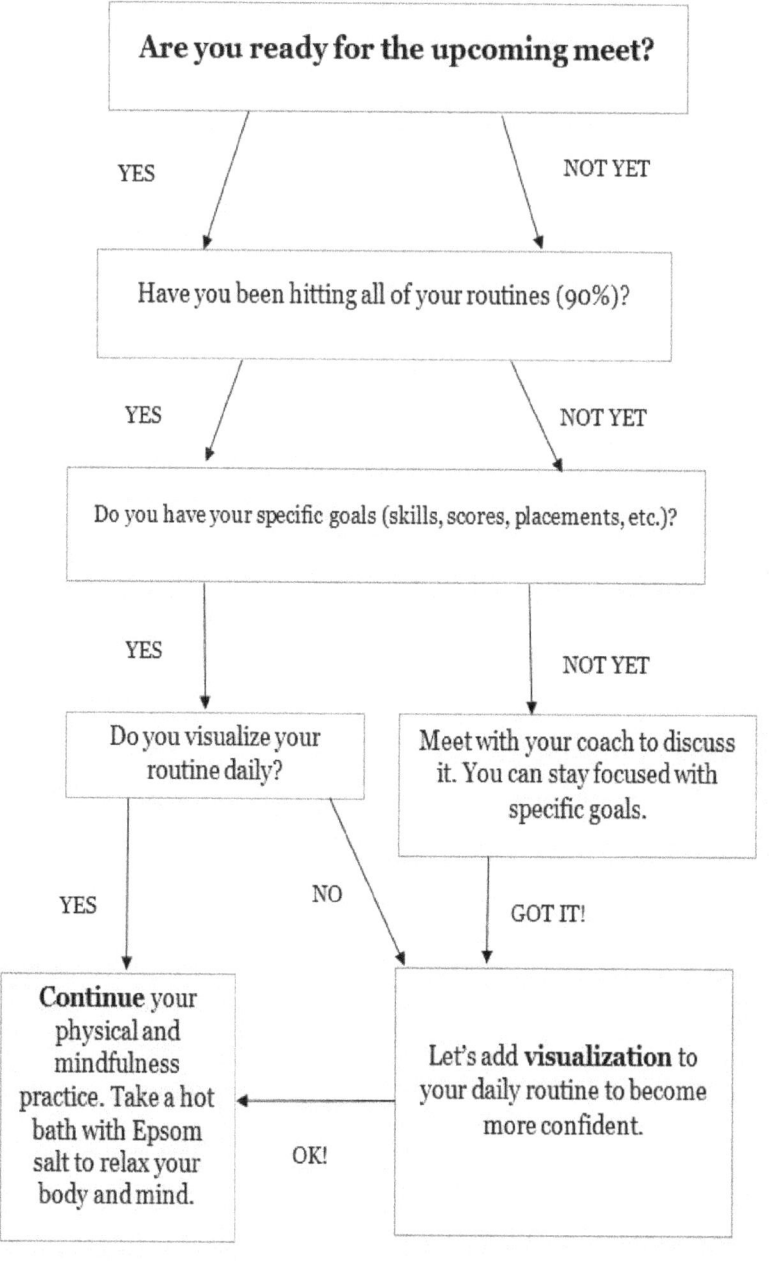

The Day of Competition: Are You Nervous?

Did I practice enough? What skills am I worried about? What if I don't place? If you notice your jumble of distracting thoughts, follow this flow chart to find your confidence.

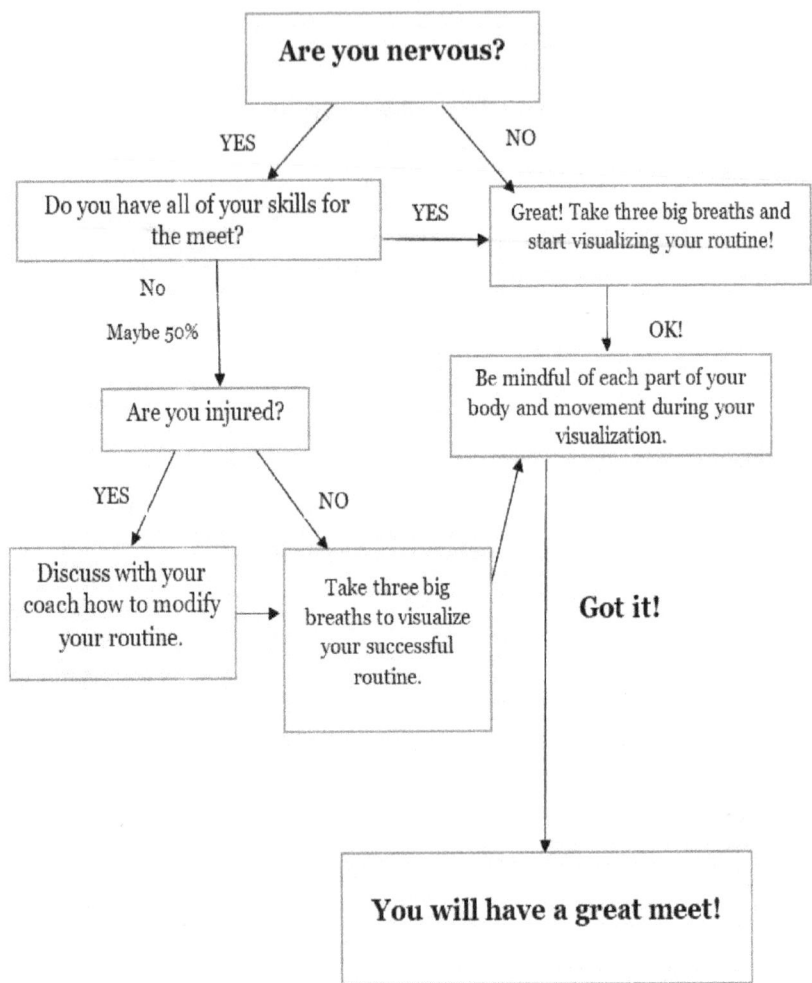

Chapter 4

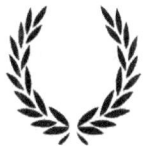

The Champion*slip* Again

Spokane, Washington, May 2019

It was the Western National Championship. Team Chelsea, including Baumpa, Nana, Baba (grandmother from Japan), Dad, and Mom, was all set. It was very unfortunate that Chelsea's brother was not able to come for this exciting event, but it was too hard to coordinate with his college exam schedule. What a great way to complete the season by being in such a big competition like this one. My husband and I felt overwhelmed and proud of how far she had come since her first injury. Whatever would happen, we were ready to congratulate her.

Thursday was the all-gymnasts practice day, grouped together by the region that they belong to. We dropped her off and let her do what she needed to do. When we picked her up, she told me that her hands had slipped from the bar. Her face was pale and tight, but she kept saying, "It's okay." At dinner, she started sobbing and said, "My shoulder hurts." Sadly, "slipping" happened to be the theme of this season. We looked for a local walk-in clinic, but instead decided to put ice on her shoulder that night and just watch how her pain might progress.

The next morning, it was not so exciting; we were all sad and worried. As a parent, you feel your child's pain as bad as she experiences it. First thing in the morning, I brought her to a walk-in acupuncturist clinic, hoping it would calm her emotional stress beyond her physical pain. I was very grateful that the competition was late enough for her to have enough time to nap and rest.

Ready or not, Chelsea wanted to do the best she could at the meet, and my job was to respect that and keep us both calm. Starting with the vault, her routine had been modified since the beginning of the season to ease the strain on her recovering elbow. She darted like a bull towards the vault, flew beautifully in the air, and landed safely. An astonishing Tsukahara. Her teammates in Region 2 cheered and clapped, especially since they all saw her slips from yesterday.

Her second event was the uneven bars. She slipped from the bar. And again. And again. After the third time, she respectfully ended her performance. My heart was racing so hard; I hoped she was okay. I tried so hard not to cry as I watched her exchange words with her coach.

My gymnast moved to the next event as if nothing had happened and started to warm up. I took a deep breath and set my phone to video to record her next performance. She saluted with a smile to the judges, and then put her hands on the floor to mount onto the beam from a unique handstand position. Chelsea gracefully turned 180 degrees, jumped with her straight splits, and shook her hips for a dance element. Then, she combined a front aerial and back flip and stuck on the beam. She picked up her vibe naturally and performed like a butterfly towards the dismount. Chelsea took one second to salute to the judges after the landing, making sure her landing was a complete stick.

As she walked off, both of her coaches approached her and gave her hugs. Her teammates and other gymnasts' coaches, too, congratulated her. Nobody could explain what they had just witnessed. We all wondered how disciplined Chelsea's mind was. I humbly announced that it was called a "master mind." Slips are part of the process that everybody must go through to become a champion. Slips are painful for any gymnast, especially in their mind. When your mind is in pain, your physical skills can be intimidated accordingly. Slips happen, so let them happen and focus on the moment, because you cannot fix your slips after you slipped.

A champion slips. But a true champion knows that slips are part of the process to becoming a champion. After all, slips don't control them. The champion controls the slips. It doesn't matter how you are placed at the meet, so define your own terms of what a champion really is to you. Is it moving up to the next level? Proceeding to the state championships, regional championships, or national championships? Being qualified as an elite? Or simply, like Chelsea, getting up strong and trying again in each practice, just because you love gymnastics? No matter what vision you have, make it clear. With your crystal clear vision, simply go back to the Resilience Cycle and take your own actions as soon as you can. When you start your own journey, it is the beginning of your own championship. Daily mindfulness practice will help you refocus on what's important when doubt and fear appear in your mind. It is powerful to notice negative emotions, but don't let them take over! Find your calm and follow the Fearless Chart to navigate your scattered mind into a focused mind. Instead of worrying about your perfect landing before tumbling, focus on the specific muscles you have to use at the moment. As long as you demonstrate your best focus each time, give yourself credit no matter how it goes. Your brain wants to think it's okay to fall because the next thing you will do is to stand back up. And each time you practice a skill, even if you fall or land it perfectly, you are getting closer to where you want to be. Falling is not failing—it is learning. When you fall, you are able to learn exactly what you need to change so you can improve. Yes, it can hurt you physically when you slip and fall, but its pain does not need to be emotional too. Don't let it stop you from loving gymnastics and becoming a champion. Let's celebrate the Champions*lips*!

Update on Chelsea, December 2019

After the 2018-2019 season was over, Chelsea's wrist, which was on the opposite side of her bad elbow, started to hurt. Who could imagine she would earn winning medals in the state, the regional, and the Western National Championships with her traumatic start in the season and her recovering elbow? We assumed that her wrist was compensating for a long time, though it was strong enough to compete in all of the events last season. While she is managing her pain and modifying her practice/routine, Chelsea decided to enjoy her beam routine as a specialist in the new competition season if her wrist continues to hurt. In addition, she rolled her ankle during the simple warmups in the optional gymnasts' clinic in early November 2019. That caused another long break from practice, although Chelsea participated in every possible conditioning exercise with her teammates. Injury is sadly common in this sport, no matter how carefully we try to prevent it. We know many of you can relate to Chelsea's ups and downs.

Please always remember, you are not alone. Instead of masking your true feelings or struggling by yourself, bring your attention to your breath. Chelsea and I believe in you as much as we do in her. So take a big breath! You can always find your own joy and purpose in gymnastics that you love.

CPSIA information can be obtained
at www.ICGtesting.com
Printed in the USA
BVHW042126281022
650574BV00003B/108